I0420646

Essential Oils for Oily Skin

Essential Oil Recipes for
Oily Skin
for Diffusers, Roller Bottles,
Inhalers & more.

Rica V. Gadi

Copyright © 2019 by The Oil Natural Empress

All rights reserved. This book or any portion thereof may not be reproduced or used in any manner whatsoever without the express written permission of the publisher except for the use of brief quotations in a book review.

Printed in the United States of America

First Printing, 2019

ISBN: 9781089780649

http://eorecipes.net

DISCLAIMER: This document is a compilation of recipes used successfully by EO enthusiasts who use only high-quality, therapeutic-grade essential oils as determined by many factors including growth, growth location, harvesting process, distillation method used, etc. Please be advised that not all essential oils are created equally, and not all essential oils are suitable for topical use or ingestion. Please do your research before choosing the brand(s) of essential oils you decide to use as well as the supplies you use. Always follow label directions on the essential oil bottles.

All the recipes in this book have been inspired by essential oil believers. However, we are not medical practitioners and do not diagnose, treat or prescribe treatment for any health condition or disease. Just a precaution, before using any alternative medicine, natural supplements, or vitamins, you should always discuss the products you are using or intend to use with your doctor, especially if you are pregnant, trying to get pregnant or nursing.

All information contained within this book is for reference purposes only, and is not intended to substitute for advice given by a pharmacist, physician or other licensed health-care professional. As such, the author is not responsible for any loss, claim or damage arising from the use of the essential oil recipes contained herein.

This book is dedicated to all the strong people who are taking responsibility for your own well being and doing something to be better.

All my heartfelt gratitude to the following people: my mom Ruby Jane, you have made me everything I am today; my dad Nestor-- my eternal, my angel, and the source of my perseverance; Mommyling, my spiritual guide ; Ria & Joe, the true witnesses of my transformation and my foundation pillars; Ellie Jane, the sparkle of our eyes;

Juan, thanks for always encouraging me to push harder - you are my ONE; Rocco & Radha, my reason for everything.

The Love of my family and friends is the fountain of inspiration that never runs dry. Thank you for constantly inspiring me, motivating me, and loving me unconditionally.

This book will never be complete without the help of my trusted and talented friends the #NOWsuperstars and my #oilbularya friends

Blending Essential Oils to use for a very specific reason has become very popular in recent years. There are several reasons why this is so. Blending EOs is basically about inhaling - as it has been proven that aromas have the ability to trigger feelings, emotions and personal memories.

With this in mind, it is obvious that everyone is unique when it comes to what triggers your senses. It all boils down to personal preference for the aroma to trigger what you want to unleash. Everyone is different and we all connect to the aroma differently, so what might work for one might not work for another person.

Of course, we also want the blend we personalize to be therapeutic. This is the best reason why to blend essential oils. We want the blend we create to help us with a very specific emotion or physical conditions. As much as smelling good is important in a blend, it is more important that we blend oils that are not only pleasing to the smell but also produces the therapeutic effect we are after.

Then you have to think about contraindications. Making sure the blend you create is safe to use.

I suggest that before blending, find out if the oils you are using are safe for a condition you may have, for example, if you are pregnant, or have specific allergies. Consult your physician prior to moving forward.

The recipes I have in this book is a compilation of what has proven to work and favored by hundreds of EO enthusiasts. It takes out the guesswork to get you started.

Again, we urge you to read the recipes and make sure that this is safe for you to try.

The book is very specific to a physical and emotional condition. There are several recipes here because you might want to rotate and you may like one and not the other. There are also a variety of applications. Some of us prefer to diffuse, some to make roller bottles, and others to create inhalers and sprays.

I hope you enjoy this compilation, feel free to use the notes section and jot down your fave blends. There is a wonderful world of EO blending - this is just the beginning.

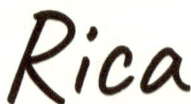

Oily skin can cause as many problems like dry skin. It happens when sebaceous glands in the body produce an excessive amount of sebum. This may cause several irritations in the face and body such as excess grease and acne. Oily skin is caused by several different factors. There are people that are naturally oily and sometimes it depends on a person's age as well. Adolescents are usually oilier because of hormonal changes. Other factors that can affect if a person has oily skin are based on location and climate. This changes how the skin adapts and produces oil in the body. Another thing that may lead to having oily skin is using the wrong skin care products or using too many skin care products.

To an extent, having oily skin can be beneficial, but too much excess can cause dirt and dead skin cells to get clogged in the skin. If an individual has larger pores, this can cause more blockages and eventually lead to acne breakouts. No one likes an uncomfortable feeling and having oily skin can be very disturbing to a person's personal and social life. There are several ways to prevent oily skin and it takes proper research and knowledge about certain products and methods to prevent it.

In most cases, oily skin can be prevented with proper skin care routines and using the right products. It is not something incredibly dangerous health-wise but having oily skin can be quite troublesome and uncomfortable. It is especially an issue for teenagers undergoing puberty. At times, having oily skin becomes the root of insecurity which is dangerous for a person's emotional and mental health.

If certain products or preventive measures to decrease oily skin have been made but it still persists, it is better to seek advice from a dermatologist. At times, trying a lot of things to remove oily skin can backfire and make it worse; therefore, having a professional's help should be taken.

Some examples of essential oils that are good for the skin is Tea tree oil. This is the most recommended essential oil for oily skin. It also has anti-inflammatory and anti-bacterial properties that prevent side effects of irritation. Another good essential oil that not many know about is Fennel essential oil. It serves as a good tonic for people with oily skin and its estrogenic properties nourish the skin and help prevent wrinkles and fine lines. This means that it encourages a healthier and more youthful-looking skin.

Table of Contents

Best Essential Oils for Oily Skin

Most experts believe that oily skin has nothing to do with a person's diet or lifestyle choices. Oily skin is the result of the sebaceous glands producing an excessive amount of oil. There are advantages to this skin type, however.

A conventional product to reduce oil may or may not contain toxic chemicals. An essential oil or an essential oil blend, on the other hand, would include none of those toxins.

Today, essential oils are used as natural oils that can contribute positively to the mind, body, and soul, and the practice is called aromatherapy. Essential oils can be used in primarily three ways. You can breathe them in, such as with an essential oil diffuser, put a few drops in the bath water, or rub them onto the skin when mixed with a carrier oil.

1. Rosemary essential oil

Rosemary essential oil comes from the rosemary plant, which is a perennial herb native to the Mediterranean region. Rosemary is an essential oil that's as popular as a lavender essential oil for its many uses, including benefitting oily skin. The oil has antiseptic and antimicrobial qualities that are good for oily skin and for reducing the spread of bacteria. It naturally rejuvenates the skin and is an excellent natural alternative to commercial toners.

2. Cedarwood Essential Oil

Cedarwood oil that is derived from the wood of cedar trees that can be found in North America. It is useful for preventing clogged pores and the spread of acne bacteria. As with almost all essential oils, you should always dilute cedarwood oil with a carrier oil, such as jojoba or olive oil. It can also be combined with other essential oils to benefit oily skin.

For example, you can combine three drops of cedarwood essential oil with two drops of tea tree oil and three drops of lavender oil. Mix this blend with four teaspoons of jojoba carrier oil. Then, apply it to the face either as a facial massage or with clean cotton balls.

3. Lemon Essential Oil

Lemon oil is extracted from the skin of the lemon. It helps to reduce blackheads and other skin pigmentation issues. Applying lemon oil directly on the affected areas helps to reduce dark spots within a week.

The best way to use lemon oil is to add it with body moisturizer as it helps to reduce the dark skin on knees and even on the elbows. It also acts as an anti-aging oil.

The best way to use lemon essential oil is by using it with a kind of facemask. Take a tbsp of gram flour mixed with curd and 2-3 drops of lemon essential oil for skin brightening. This facemask gives an instant glow and freshness on an oily face for at least 4-5 hours of applying. And regularly using it helps to reduce acne scars and other skin pigmentation.

4. Grapeseed Essential Oil

I learned more about grapeseed oil after using Plum Buckthorn oil, which contains ten oils benefits. Let me tell you grapeseed oil is also extracted from the seed of grapes. It is enriched with omega 3 and other fatty acids which make the skin glow from inside. It also contains a high amount of Vitamin C, D, and E.

Grapeseed oil is mostly used to reduce wrinkles and acne scars. Most of the essential oils available in the market contain grapeseed oil which helps to control skin aging. It does tighten the skin and moisturizes the skin from deep inside. And mostly this oil does not block the sebaceous gland and does not cause acne.

Massaging your skin regularly with grapeseed during night time skincare routine helps to restore glow and controls aging.

5. Ylang Ylang Essential Oil

If you have oily and acne prone skin, Ylang Ylang oil is your skin savior. Not only it fights acne; at the same time, it also retains the moisture of the skin. It balances sebum production and also relieves skin from the blemishes. If you're suffering from adult acne, this oil can help you get rid of it!

This oil suits a variety of skin types especially the combination, oily and acne prone skin. Did you know that it has anti-aging ingredients which reduces fine lines and improve skin elasticity.

6. Geranium Essential Oil

This essential oil may not be as well-known as lavender or tea tree, but its properties are suitable for regulating sebum production and reducing the appearance of oily skin, as well as healing acne scars. Geranium essential oil comes from the Pelargonium species or the leaves of the geranium plant. This is an essential oil that can be used as a natural astringent.

7. Tea Tree Essential Oil

One of the best essential oils for oily skin is melaleuca oil, also known as tea tree oil. This is an oil derived from the tea tree, a multi-trunked tree found in Australia. You will see that the oil is especially popular these days, especially in places where massage therapists practice.

What's great about this oil is that it has antibacterial properties, which are ideal for treating conditions such as pimples and acne, common with oily skin. This is a potent oil that should always be diluted with a carrier oil to avoid allergic skin reactions and should not be ingested.

The Blending Process

These EOs are categorized by aromas, and EOs from the same group usually blend fantastically together.

- Floral – Lavender, Geranium, Jasmine
- Woodsy – Pine, Cedarwood
- Earthy – Vetiver, Patchouli
- Herbaceous – Marjoram, Rosemary, Basil
- Minty – Peppermint, Spearmint, Wintergreen
- Medicinal – Eucalyptus, Frankincense, Melaleuca
- Spicy – Pepper, Clove, Cinnamon
- Oriental – Ginger, Patchouli
- Citrus – Wild Orange, Lemon, Lime

Select oils that will give you the health benefits you are looking to remedy. For increased energy choose: Grapefruit, Lemon, Orange, or Citrus. For Calming and Relaxation choose: Lavender, Cedarwood, or Chamomile. You are encouraged to experiment and play with your oils to see which blends work for you.

TIPS:

- Combine Floral EOs with Woodsy, Spicy and Citrus aromas
- Minty EOs with Woodsy, Earthy, Herbaceous and Citrus aromas
- Earthy EOs with Woodsy and Minty aromas
- Citrus EOs with Floral, Woodsy, Minty, Spicy and Oriental aromas

Essential Oils Substitution List

Sometimes we want to blend oils but we just don't have all the oils as stated in a recipe. I've created an easy to use guide for substitution.

Name of Oil	SUB 1	SUB 2	SUB 3
Arborvitae	Melissa	Cedarwood	Patchouli
Basil	Massage Blend	Marjoram	Thyme
Bergamot	Grapefruit	Lime	
Birch	Wintergreen	Cypress	
Black Pepper	Copaiba	Juniper Berry	Clove
Blue Tansy	Roman Chamomile		
Cardamom	Lavender	Clary Sage	Roman Chamomile
Cassia	Cinnamon		
Cedarwood	Arborvitae	Patchouli	Vetiver
Cellular Blend	Frankincense	Thyme	Clove
Cilantro	Coriander	Cardamom	Black Pepper
Cinnamon	Cassia		
Clary Sage	Ylang Ylang		
Clove	Cassia	Cinnamon	
Copaiba	Thyme	Oregano	Clove
Coriander	Lavender	Juniper Berry	Cardamom

Cypress	Douglas Fir	Massage Blend	Copaiba
Detoxification Blend	Geranium	Copaiba	Rosemary
Digestive Blend	Fennel	Peppermint	Ginger
Dill	Bergamot	Lemon	Wild Orange
Douglas Fir	Siberian Fir	Cypress	
Eucalyptus	Respiratory Blend	Melaleuca	Melissa
Frankincense	Cedarwood		
Geranium	Copaiba	Rose	
Ginger	Digestive Blend	Fennel	Geranium
Grapefruit	Bergamot	Lemon	Wild Orange
Helichrysum	Myrrh		
Jasmine	Roman Chamomile	Rose	Ylang Ylang
Juniper Berry	Coriander		
Lavender	Petitgrain	Roman Chamomile	Coriander
Lemon	Wild Orange	Lime	Grapefruit
Lemongrass	Helichrysum	Cilantro	
Marjoram	Basil	Cypress	
Melaleuca	Neroli	Rosemary	Eucalyptus
Melissa	Black Pepper	Eucalyptus	

Metabolic Blend	Ginger	Peppermint	Cinnamon
Myrrh	Sandalwood	Spikenard	
Neroli	Rosemary	Melissa	Melaleuca
Oregano	Thyme	Basil	Copaiba
Patchouli	Vetiver	Focus Blend	Cedarwood
Peppermint	Spearmint		
Petitgrain	Lavender	Wild Orange	Bergamot
Protective Blend	Cinnamon	Clove	Copaiba
Renewing Blend	Bergamot	Juniper Berry	Myrrh
Respiratory Blend	Eucalyptus	Rosemary	Melaleuca
Roman Chamomile	Blue Tansy	Lavender	Focus Blend
Rose	Geranium	Jasmine	Ylang Ylang
Rosemary	Melaleuca	Neroli	Eucalyptus
SandalWood	Cedarwood	Spikenard	Myrrh
Siberian Fir	Douglas Fir	White Fir	Cedarwood
Soothing Blend	Helichrysum	Peppermint	Wintergreen
Spearmint	Peppermint	Reassuring Blend	
Spikenard	Myrrh	Vetiver	Patchouli
Thyme	Oregano	Copaiba	Clove

Vetiver	Patchouli	Spikenard	Cedarwood
White Fir	Siberian Fir	Douglas Fir	
Wild Orange	Tangerine	Lemon	Grapefruit
Wintergreen	Birch	Siberian Fir	
Ylang Ylang	Jasmine	Lavender	

Diffuse

Diffusing Essential Oils is the safest
method to enjoy Essential Oils
without the risk of an allergic reaction.

Diffusing Essential Oils
Some Tidbits You Need To Know

Our sense of smell is one of our most powerful senses, and as you have noticed in your own experience, some scents affect you more positively in your minds than others. The body contains over 1,000 receptors for smell—way more receptors than for any of our other senses.

Diffusion Essential Oils means the process vaporizes oils into the air by releasing tiny amounts into the air. Inhalation is totally safe and is super low risk. Chances of any EO rising to dangerous levels while diffusion is slim to none.

Diffusing Essential Oils around newborns, babies, young children, pregnant or nursing women, and pets should be done with caution. Read up on safety.

It is advisable that Diffusing Essential Oils for only about 15-30 minutes at a time to be most effective. NEVER leave your diffuser on overnight. Make sure your diffuser is filled with the right amount of water and you understand the operating directions.

While diffusing essential oils, be sure that your space has great ventilation. Crack a window open if the scent becomes strong.

Never add Carrier Oils to your diffuser. This may cause your diffuser to malfunction. Clean your diffuser at least 3 times a week with warm water and natural soap to ensure the diffuser is well maintained and bacteria and mold does not accumulate.

Diffusing Essential Oils
Basic Guidelines

Just a few things you need to know and prepare before getting started Diffusing Essential Oils.

Things you need:
Ultrasonic Oil Diffuser
Essential Oils
Water

Just follow the number of drops in the recipe, drop on to an oil diffuser and fill the rest with water.

All diffusers are different and will have its own water minimum and maximum level. Read the diffuser instruction before use.

Ideally, it is best to diffuse for 15-30 minutes and turn off the diffuser. The effect should be good for at least 2-3 hours. Turn your diffuser back on after 3 hours to reinforce oil diffusing effects.

It is not advisable to use EO in humidifiers.

These are not made to release EOS

Roll

Essential Oil Roller Bottles is the easiest method to enjoy Essential Oils Anywhere and Whenever.

Blending Essential Oils in a Roller Bottle
Some Tidbits You Need To Know

Essential Oils are usually super concentrated and too hard to measure how much to actually put straight from the bottle.

Roller bottles are a way that you are able to create blends ready to use with the right dilution. It allows your EO to last longer.

It also makes it easier to apply exactly where you want to target without getting it all over the place.

It is handy and easy to carry in your purse, ready to use at any time you want to.

I like to apply EOs at the bottom of the feet for many reasons. Our feet have bigger pores than any other skin in our bodies. This means that they are able to suck in the therapeutic compounds in our blend into the bloodstream faster than any other parts of the body. Imagine comparing a normal straw to an oversized straw and how much more you can suck in with the latter. This is how the soles of our feet are compared to the rest of the skin in our bodies.

The skin on our feet is also less sensitive and is designed to withstand some abuse. The risk of having an irritation from EOS is less likely to happen when applied on the feet.

The feet don't have the glands that act as a barrier. Sebaceous glands are glands in our skin that produce an oily substance called Sebum, for the purpose of lubricating and waterproofing the skin. Since this is oil and if you put oil on top of oil, it can act as a barrier or it may slow down penetration.

The feet and palms of our hands are the only skin that don't have these, so it is ideal to apply Essential Oils to the feet for maximum penetration.

Now, it would be hard to apply oils directly and very messy, right? Roller bottles make it super easy and convenient to roll the EOs at the bottom of our feet.

Carrier Oils Info

Carrier oils are vegetable-based oils with their own healing properties that dilute essential oils used to help carry the EOs into the skin.

Essential oils are highly concentrated and could evaporate very quickly. The carrier oil is mixed with the essential oil so it could penetrate the skin before it actually evaporates. Although EOs are oils, it is actually not that oily. When mixed with a carrier oil, it allows you to have more of the essential oil into your skin without wasting EOS to evaporate, making the healing properties of the EO strong and more effective.

There are also Essential oils that are too strong to apply directly to the skin and may cause damage, so it is important to dilute them with carrier oil.

Never add Carrier Oils to your diffuser. This may cause your diffuser to malfunction. Clean your diffuser at least 3 times a week with warm water and natural soap to ensure the diffuser is well maintained and bacteria and mold does not accumulate.

Carrier Oils

There are a lot of different carrier oils that you can use with EOs to dilute them in a roller bottle.

To name a few :

Almond Oil - moisturizing and stays liquid at room temperature. Do not use it if you are allergic to nuts.

Apricot Kernel Oil - moisturizing and suitable for sensitive skin or kids. It is super gentle on the skin.

Avocado Oil - moisturizing and suitable for sensitive and damaged skin. Perfect for skin problems.Can be mixed with other carrier oils

Castor Oil - with antibacterial, antiviral and antifungal properties, use topically to eliminate pain and relieve skin irritation.

Coconut Oil - its antibacterial, antiviral and antifungal properties it is the best and most versatile for skin care. The skin absorbs this very quickly. It solidifies in room temp and may still have a slight coconut oil aroma in it - but you can get fractionated coconut oil to eliminate the 2 challenges above.

Grapeseed Oil - not just for cooking but also great for topical application on the skin.

Jojoba Oil - one of my faves for skin care blends. This oil is the closest to our natural oil our skin produces so it is absorbed easily without being oily. Also amazing for massage oil blends.

Olive Oil - this is the oil for herb type oils. mostly used for cooking but can also be applied to the skin but would need to be blended with a carrier oil that is mild and absorb well with the skin.

Rosehip Seed Oil - super good for deep moisturizing or skin irritations. This oil has a high content of antioxidants and helps remedy dry, scarred and wounded skin.

Recommended Roller Bottle Dilution Guide

RECOMMENDED ROLL-ON BOTTLE DILUTION AMOUNTS

5 ml (1/6 oz.) Roll-on Bottle = ~100 drops (1tsp.)
10 ml (1/3 oz.) Roll-on Bottle = ~200 drops (2 tsp.)
30 ml. (1 oz.) Roll-on Bottle = ~600 drops (6 tsp.)

Roll-on Size	5 ml	10 ml	30 ml	Add EO drops to roll-on, then fill with carrier oil.	
Essential Oil Drops	1	2	6	1%	Dilution Percentage
	2	4	12	2%	
	3	6	18	3%	
	5	10	30	5%	
	10	20	60	10%	
	20	40	120	20%	
	25	50	150	25%	
	50	100	300	50%	

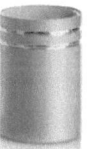

General Guidelines:
Birth to 12 months = .3-.5% dilution
1-5 years = 1.5-3% dilution
6-11 years = 1.5-5% dilution
12-17 years = 1.5-20% dilution
18 years and older = 1.5% dilution-Neat (no dilution)
Elderly or Sensitive Skin = 1-3% dilution
Daily Use = 2-5% dilution
Short Term Use = 10-25% dilution
Local Skin or Systemic Issues = 50% dilution-Neat

*These are general guidelines suggestions--not absolute rules--based on traditional aromatheraphy practice.
(Kurt Schnaubelt PhD, Valerie Worwood, Robert Tisserand)*

Dilution Basics:

How much you dilute your EO depends on different factors such as weight, sensitivity, health conditions, EOs that are blended in or how long that blend has been used for. There is never an absolute dilution rule, it is you who knows about your level and tolerance. I feel that it is best to start with a higher dilution percentage and increase EO drops over time.

To make sure your EO is safe, make sure that the oils you use are therapeutic grade and do your research on the source and extraction methods used to produce the oils.

Roller Bottle Blending Order

I normally just start with dropping the drops of oil into the **10mL roller bottle**, then adding the carrier oil up until the shoulder of the bottle. Capping the bottle off with the roller and the bottle cap. Instead of shaking the bottle, I like to roll the bottle between my palms first for a minute or 2 for blending, then finishing it off with a few shakes.

NOTE: All recipes in this book are for a 10mL Roller Bottle. If you have a bigger or smaller roller bottle, adjust the number of EO drops based on the size of your bottle.

Inhale

Essential Oil Inhalers are the most convenient way to enjoy Essential Oils Anywhere and Whenever.

Essential Oil Inhalers give you quick and easy access to the vast therapeutic benefits of essential oils.

Blending Essential Oils in an Inhaler
Some Tidbits You Need To Know

EO Inhalers or aroma sticks are compact tubes, with a cotton wick inside and a protective cover, to lock the aroma within.

Your preferred blend of essential oils is absorbed by the cotton wick, and safely enclosed in a tube that fits inside of the cover. The cover is easily removed for access to the tube to breathe in the aroma. Usually lasts about 3 months, depending on the oil blend used.

I absolutely love these because they encourage me to take a moment during super stressful moments, and just breathe.

It is in times of stress when our breathing patterns often change and taking deep breaths promote a feeling of calm and inner peace. Breath work combined with visualization plus a relaxing inhaler, can offer relief to symptoms of stress and help your body to come back to the state of homeostasis.

Aroma Sticks can be carried in your tiny purse, even compact enough to fit in your pocket. You can enjoy your favorite EOs anywhere and you can use them with discretion.

I love diffusing, and do all the time but not everyone in my space may enjoy the scents I enjoy or they may not benefit from the therapeutic benefits of the EOs I am diffusing - so the inhaler is one way to not only enjoy my choice of blends but to keep in personal not affecting everyone else around me.

Inhalers not only benefits me but also keep those around me safe in case the oils I want to blend may pose a risk to those around me who may have a health issue not advised to be exposed to my choice EOs/

When making Aroma Sticks, You may use your chosen EOs at 100% Concentration.

Inhaler Basic Guidelines

Breathe in slow and deep to absorb the EO molecules directly into your olfactory system.

Inhalers are super easy to use. You just remove the cap and inhale from the inhaler tube, count 1 to 5 slowly as you inhale. The EO molecules get drawn into our bloodstream through our nasal cavity and get delivered throughout our entire body.

Simple to use, easy to carry, portable and compact. You never have to be without your favorite blends, ever.

Inhaler Blending Basics

Inhalers are super easy and simple to make.

All you need is an inhaler set which consist of the following:

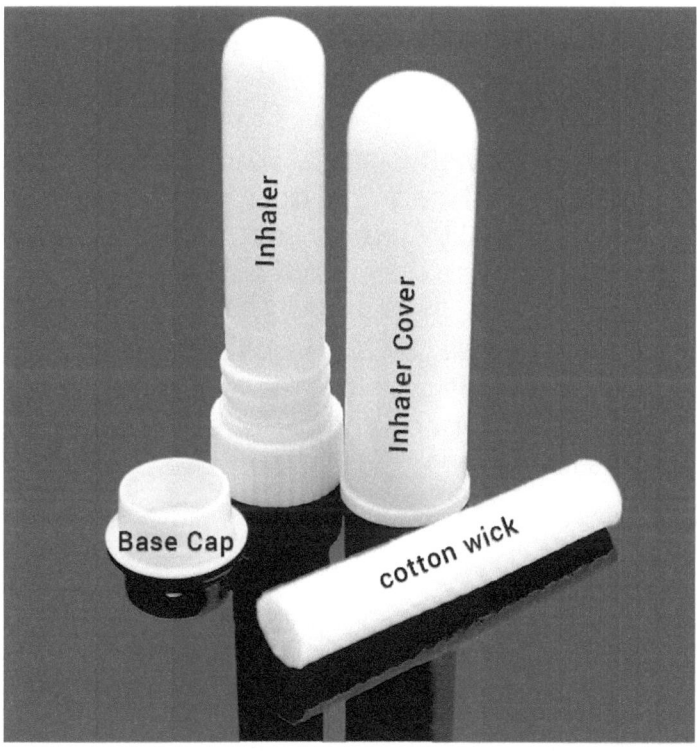

Inhaler, Inhaler Cover, Base Cap and Cotton Wick.

You will need your Essential Oils.

I like to use a pipette for precision and a small petri dish so I can see the oil.

Blending is super easy, just combine the drops and swirl it around in the petri dish and when you are satisfied you can go ahead and drop the cotton wick to absorb all the oil in the dish.

Once the wick is ready you can drop it in the inhaler and cap the bottom with the Base Cap. I usually like to secure the cover with the inhaler so I don't have to do it later.

I usually use 15-20 drops of EO total in a recipe and it can last up to 3 months. Some recipes will need more but on average it is in this range.

EO Recipes for Oily Skin

DIY Hydrating Face Oil

3 tbsp Jojoba oil
1 ½ tbsp Argan oil
2 tsp Rosehip Seed oil
1/4 tsp Vitamin E
4 drops Carrot Seed
8 drops Geranium
2 oz. Dark dropper bottle

Pour all the ingredients into a dropper bottle.
Shake before use.
Cleanse your face. Apply toner.
Gently massage about a ¼ to ½ dropper full of oil blend onto your face and neck.

Aloe Vera Jelly and Honey Face Mask

2 drops Lavender
1 drop Lemon
1 drop Cypress
2 tbsp Aloe Vera Jelly
1 tbsp Honey

Mix Aloe Vera Jelly and essential oils, then mix with honey.
Apply to the face, avoiding the eye area.
Let it for 15-30 minutes.
Wash off with lukewarm water and pat dry.
Re-apply 2 times a week.

Sugar Face Scrub

2 tsp Sunflower Carrier Oil
3 drops Orange
2 tsp Honey
2 tsp Brown Sugar (more or less for your
desired consistency)

Pour the Sunflower Carrier Oil, Orange and
Honey into a bowl and make sure that it is
well mixed.
Then, add the sugar (keep adding sugar
until the mixture has a consistency that is
gritty enough to scrub your skin, but still wet
enough to apply it easily).
Apply the scrub to a freshly washed face, rub
the scrub all over your face.
Wash off with water and pat dry.

DIY All-Natural Face Oil for Acne-Prone & Oily Skin

3 tablespoons Jojoba oil
1 tablespoon Tamanu oil
6 drops Lavender
6 drops Frankincense

Add all the ingredients to the dropper bottle.
Put the cap on and shake the bottle.
Apply 4-6 drops to clean, dry skin.

Vanilla Lotion

1/2 cup Almond oil or Jojoba oil (or any other liquid oil)
1/4 cup Coconut oil
1/4 cup Beeswax
1 tsp Vitamin E oil (optional)
2 tbsp Shea Butter or Cocoa Butter (optional)
2 drops Essential oil or Vanilla extract

Combine the oils, butter with the wax in a double boiler. As they melt, stir and let it cool off. Add vitamin E oil and pour it into a jar of your choice.

DIY Blackhead Removal Mask

1 tbsp Gelatin
1 drop Peppermint Essential Oil
1 drop Frankincense Essential Oil
½ tsp Turmeric

Heap up 1/8 cup of water in a pan and when warm, place the water in a small dish.
Stir and add the peppermint essential oil.
Blend well the gelatin.
Stir and add frankincense essential oil.
Apply to your entire face and neck.
Dry and gently peel it off.
Rinse with warm water.

DIY Coconut & Tea Tree Oil Face Scrub

2 tbsp Coconut Oil
2 tsp Organic Raw Honey
4 tbsp Organic Coffee Grounds
8 drops Carrot Seed Oil
6 drops Tea Tree Essential Oil

Blend the honey and coconut oil into a small container.
Add the coffee grounds and blend.
Add the tea tree oil and carrot seed oil.
Mix all the ingredients together.
Store mixture in the fridge, contain it in a small jar.

DIY Hydrating Face Oil

3 tbsp Jojoba Oil
1 ½ tbsp Argan Oil
2 tsp Rosehip Seed Oil
1/4 tsp Vitamin E
4 drops Carrot Seed Essential Oil
8 drops Geranium Essential Oil
2 oz. Dark Dropper Bottle

Pour into a dropper bottle the jojoba oil.
Put into the bottle the vitamin E, rosehip
seed oil and argan oil.
Blend also the carrot oil and geranium oil.
Close the lid and shake well.
To use: Clean your face, apply toner and
gently massage the oil blend into your face
and neck.

DIY Face Serum with Essential Oil

2 oz. of Carrier Oil of your choice (Jojoba, Argan Oil, Grapeseed Oil)
20 drops Essential Oil (Frankincense, Geranium, Lavender, Patchouli, Tea Tree, Ylang Ylang, Clary Sage, Roman Chamomile, Cypress, Peppermint, Rosemary, Sandalwood)
glass bottle

Pour the carrier oil into a glass bottle.
Add 20 drops of essential oils.
Mix and roll the bottle in your hand.
To use: Cleanse face, use a toner, apply a drop of your mixture serum to your face, gently massage soft upward strokes.
To store: Store in a dark and cool place.

Body Scrub Essential Oils

1 cup of Exfoliant of your choice(Salt, Sugar, Ground Coffee and Oatmeal)
1/3 cup of Macadamia Nut Oil
8 drops Sandalwood
6 drops Lemon
6 drops Lavender

Blend the macadamia nut oil into a small container.
Add the exfoliant of your choice and blend.
Add the essential oils.
Mix all the ingredients together.

Beeswax Moisturizer

¼ cup Beeswax Pellets
½ cup Coconut Oil
½ cup Olive Oil
10 drops Essential Oil (patchouli, Roman chamomile, vanilla, sandalwood, frankincense, clary sage, lavender, or geranium oil)

Utilize a twofold heater to dissolve the beeswax.
When it liquefies, expel it from the kettle and let it cool.
Include the coconut and olive oils and whip well.
Include the fundamental oil(s).
Whip the blend well until you get a rich surface.
Move the blend to a glass container and store it in a cool and dry spot (don't refrigerate).

Geranium Moisturizer

1 tsp Chamomile Tea (or dried chamomile flowers)
½ cup Water
1 tbsp Lanolin
1 tbsp Beeswax
½ cup Sweet Almond Oil
1 Vitamin A Capsule
1 Vitamin E Capsule
3 drops Geranium Essential Oil

Liquefy the shea spread in a twofold boiler. When it has mellowed, expel it from the warmth.
Include avocado oil and blend.
Include the fundamental oils and whip the blend well until it builds up a velvety surface.
Store it in a glass container and use it as your everyday face cream.

Chamomile Toner

2 drops Camphor Oil
2 drops Chamomile Oil
1 tbsp Rose Water

Put all the ingredients in a glass bowl and mix them well.
Soak a cotton ball in the toner and gently apply it all over the dry skin on your face and neck.
You can use it once every two weeks to revitalize dry skin.

DIY All-Natural Face Oil for Acne-Prone & Oily Skin

3 tbsp Jojoba Oil
1 tsp Tamanu oil
6 drops Lavender
6 drops Frankincense

Add all the ingredients to the dropper bottle.
Put the cap on and shake the bottle.
Apply 4-6 drops to clean, dry skin.

Chamomile Body Spray

1 oz Helichrysum Hydrosol
1 oz Rose water Hydrosol
1 oz Chamomile Hydrosol
1 oz Lavender Hydrosol
1 drop Lavender Essential Oil
1 drop Chamomile Essential Oil

Mix all the recipes in a dim, 4-ounce glass
spray container.
Splash onto dry skin day and night following
purifying.

Sandalwood Mask

2 tbsp Clay (bentonite, green and white all work)
2 tsp Cornstarch
2 tsp Raw Honey
1 tsp Evening Primrose Oil or Rose-hip Seed oil
1 Egg Yolk
2 drops Rose
2 drops Lavender
2 drops Sandalwood

Mix ingredients together.
Apply to skin and leave on for 15 minutes.
Rinse off with cool water.

Myrrh Moisturizer

3 tbsp Shea Butter
1 tsp Vitamin E Oil
1 tsp Aloe Vera Gel
3 tbsp Apricot Seed Oil
5 drops Helichrysum Essential Oil
5 drops Myrrh Essential Oil
3 drops Clary Sage Essential Oil

Liquefy the shea spread in a twofold heater and enable it to chill off a bit.
Whisk the spread once it chills off and includes oils and aloe vera gel. Continue blending.
When it arrives at a smooth consistency, move the cream to a glass compartment.
Apply it to your face and body as and when required.

Your Own EO Blends

Your Own EO Blends

Book Ordering

To order your copy / copies of
Essential Oils
for Oily Skin

please visit: **EOrecipes.net**

You can also check out other titles available.

Bulk Pricing and
Affiliate Programs Available

www.ingramcontent.com/pod-product-compliance
Lightning Source LLC
Chambersburg PA
CBHW021548290526
45784CB00016B/2455